AF731049

MEDICAL THINGS EXPLAINED

MTE

by Stacie the PA

Osteoporosis 101:

The Complete Patient's Guide to Prevention, Treatment and Recovery

By Stacie the PA

© 2025 Stacie Seeram, PA-C
All rights reserved.

No part of this publication may be reproduced, distributed, or transmitted in any form or by any means, including photocopying, recording, or other electronic or mechanical methods, without the prior written permission of the author, except in the case of brief quotations used in reviews or educational materials.

For permission requests, contact:
Medical Things Explained
Email: medicalthingsexplained@gmail.com

ISBN: (to be inserted after registration)
Printed in the United States of America
First Edition, 2025

Cover design and layout by Stacie the PA™
Published by Medical Things Explained/Stacie the PA/Bowker

DISCLAIMER PAGE

This book is for **educational purposes only** and is not intended to replace professional medical advice, diagnosis, or treatment.
Always seek the advice of your physician or other qualified healthcare provider with any questions you may have regarding a medical condition.

Never disregard professional medical advice or delay seeking it because of something you have read in this book.
If you think you may have a medical emergency, call your healthcare provider or local emergency number immediately.

Medication names, brand names, and supplement examples are included for patient understanding only and do not represent endorsement by the author.
Readers should consult their healthcare team before beginning any new treatment, supplement, exercise program, or lifestyle change.

Some links or products mentioned may appear on the author's Amazon page as part of an affiliate partnership. If a purchase is made through those links, the author may receive a small commission at no additional cost to the reader.

Acknowledgments & Dedication

I would like to extend my heartfelt gratitude to the many healthcare professionals I have had the privilege of working with over the past two decades. From teachers and professors who laid the foundation of my medical education to the clinicians and support teams who bring compassion and excellence to patient care every day—you have each contributed to this work in meaningful ways.

To my colleagues in medicine—physicians, physician assistants, nurse practitioners, nurses, anesthetists, pharmacists, therapists, social workers, and medical assistants—thank you for your expertise, mentorship, and shared commitment to helping patients heal and thrive. To the administrative staff, technicians, and countless behind-the-scenes professionals who make quality care possible, your work is deeply valued and never unseen.

Your collaboration, teaching, and dedication have shaped not only my career but also the clarity and empathy that guide these books. Each lesson learned, each patient helped, and each conversation shared has strengthened my belief that education is one of the most powerful tools in healthcare.

This book—and the entire 101 Series—is dedicated to all of you who continue to serve, teach, and lead with heart. Thank you for inspiring me to make medicine more understandable, more compassionate, and more human.

*A special thank-you to **Dr. Wade**, whose vision for a comprehensive Bone Health Clinic and encouragement to create this resource helped bring Osteoporosis 101 to life. Her dedication to preventive care and patient education represents exactly what this book stands for—empowering patients to take an active role in their health at every age.*

Osteoporosis affects us all, directly or indirectly—our patients, parents, grandparents, and even ourselves. May this work serve as a reminder that stronger bones begin with stronger knowledge, and that awareness, prevention, and compassion can truly change lives.

TABLE OF CONTENTS

Section 1

Introduction

What does it mean?

What Is Osteoporosis?

Osteoporosis means "porous bone."
It's a condition where bones become thin, weak, and more likely to break. Think of a healthy bone as a solid, honeycomb-like structure. With osteoporosis, those holes inside the bone get larger, and the outer walls become thinner. This makes the bone fragile—like a sponge that's lost its firmness.

Osteoporosis can happen to anyone, but it's most common in women after menopause and in older adults of both sexes. It develops slowly over many years, often without any symptoms until a fracture occurs. That's why it's sometimes called **"the silent bone disease."**

Why Does It Matter?

Strong bones help us stay active, independent, and pain-free. When bones weaken, even a small fall or simple movement—like bending or coughing—can cause a fracture.
Fractures in the hip, spine, or wrist can lead to serious problems, such as long recovery times, loss of mobility, or needing help with daily activities.

For example:

- **Hip fractures** often require surgery and can make walking or living alone difficult.
- **Spine fractures** may cause back pain, height loss, or a stooped posture.
- **Wrist fractures** can limit hand use and independence.

Preventing these injuries means protecting your bones long before a fracture happens.

Who Gets Osteoporosis?

Osteoporosis doesn't just affect "little old ladies."

- **Women** are at higher risk after menopause, when estrogen levels drop.
- **Men** can also develop it—especially if they have low testosterone or long-term medical issues.
- **Younger adults** may develop low bone mass (osteopenia) if they take certain medicines, have digestive disorders, or don't get enough calcium or vitamin D.

No matter your age, you can take steps to strengthen your bones and lower your risk.

Osteopenia vs. Osteoporosis

You may hear your provider mention **osteopenia**—this means your bone density is lower than normal but not yet in the osteoporosis range.
Osteopenia is a **warning sign.** It's the perfect time to act with diet, exercise, and healthy habits to keep bones from weakening further.

The Good News

Osteoporosis can be **managed—and often prevented.**
Today's treatments, including lifestyle changes, medications, and nutrition, can slow bone loss and even rebuild some strength. The earlier you know your risk, the more options you have.

What You'll Learn in This Book

In the chapters ahead, you'll discover:

- How bones grow and change through life
- Why bone loss happens and how to spot it early
- What tests and lab work check bone strength
- Which medications and supplements may help
- How to eat, move, and live to protect your bones
- What to expect if you do have a fracture
- And how to stay strong, steady, and independent at any age

A Message of Encouragement

Learning about osteoporosis is not about fear—it's about empowerment.
Your bones are living tissue, constantly renewing themselves. With the right care, they can stay strong for decades. This book will guide you step-by-step so you can make confident, informed choices about your bone health.

What This Book Will and Won't Do

- **What it WILL do:** give you clear steps to protect your bones, the questions to ask, and the habits that help.
- **What it WON'T do:** replace your medical provider. Big changes—new pills, new exercises, or stopping a medicine—should be done **with** your provider.
- **Your action today:** put this book with your medication list. Bring both to your next visit.

Section 2

Understanding Normal Bones

Knowing what normal means, will help with the rest

Understanding Normal Bones:

Your Bones Are Alive

Many people think of bones as hard, lifeless sticks that never change — but that's not true.
Your bones are living tissue. They are constantly breaking down old bone and rebuilding new bone in a process called **remodeling.**

Think of it like a construction crew:

- **Old bone** is broken down by cells called *osteoclasts.*
- **New bone** is built by cells called *osteoblasts.*

This remodeling happens all the time, every single day, to keep your bones strong and healthy.

How Bones Grow and Change

From birth through your teenage years, bones grow quickly in length and strength. During this time, your body is building its **bone bank** — the more "bone savings" you store when you're young, the stronger your skeleton will be later in life.

- Most people reach their **peak bone mass** — the strongest their bones will ever be — by their **late 20s.**
- After that, bone building slows down a little.
- Around **midlife**, the balance starts to shift. Your body may break down bone faster than it rebuilds it.

- After **menopause**, when estrogen levels drop, women can lose bone more quickly.
- Men also lose bone as testosterone levels decrease with age, but usually at a slower rate.

What Healthy Bone Looks Like

Healthy bone looks like a honeycomb when seen under a microscope — firm, dense, and evenly spaced.
Each little "hole" in that honeycomb helps bones stay strong but slightly flexible so they don't break easily.

When osteoporosis develops, the spaces inside that honeycomb get **larger** and the outer walls get **thinner.**
That means the bone becomes weaker and more likely to break — especially in the hip, spine, and wrist.

Quick Visual Tip:
Imagine a brand-new sponge (healthy bone) — soft but springy, full of tiny holes.
Now imagine an old, worn-out sponge — dry, thin, and full of big gaps.
That's what osteoporosis does to bone over time.

The Building Blocks of Strong Bones

Your bones need the right ingredients to stay strong, just like a house needs solid materials:

Bone Ingredient	What It Does	Where You Get It
Calcium	Main mineral that hardens bone	Dairy, leafy greens, fortified foods, supplements
Vitamin D	Helps your body absorb calcium	Sunlight, fish, eggs, fortified milk
Protein	Builds the collagen “framework” inside bones	Meat, beans, nuts, dairy, soy
Magnesium, phosphorus, vitamin K	Support bone structure and balance	Whole grains, veggies, nuts, and seeds

Without these nutrients, even strong bones can become fragile.

Why Bone Health Changes Over Time

Several things can speed up bone loss:

- **Hormone changes:** Lower estrogen or testosterone speeds bone breakdown.
- **Inactivity:** Bones stay strong when used. If you stop moving, they lose density.
- **Poor nutrition:** Too little calcium or vitamin D weakens bone over time.
- **Medications or illnesses:** Some medicines and conditions affect how bones rebuild.

Even though bone loss happens naturally with age, there's **a lot you can do** to slow it down — and even strengthen your bones again.

The Takeaway

- Your bones are alive and constantly changing.
- Strong bones come from good "bone building" when you're young and smart choices as you age.
- It's never too late to improve your bone health.
- The rest of this book will show you **how to protect, nourish, and strengthen your bones** at every stage of life.

Everyday Bone-Strengthening Habits

- You don't need a gym or special equipment to start improving your bone strength.
- Small movements, done regularly, can make a big difference.
- Here are some simple ways to build balance, muscle, and bone strength throughout your day.

Morning Routine

- **While brushing your teeth:** Stand on one leg for 30 seconds (hold the counter if needed). Switch legs the next time.
- **While getting dressed:** Try putting on pants or socks while standing (only if stable). This helps with balance and coordination.
- **When pouring coffee:** Do 5 mini calf raises — rise onto your toes, hold for a second, and lower slowly.

During the Day

- **When waiting for the microwave or kettle:** Do 10 squats or heel lifts.
- **While talking on the phone:** Walk around instead of sitting still.
- **When reaching for items in the cabinet:** Use your core — stand tall, tighten your stomach muscles, and avoid twisting quickly.
- **At your desk:** Every 30 minutes, stand up and stretch your arms overhead or do gentle side bends.

Around the House

- **Laundry time:** Use detergent bottles or gallon jugs as light weights — lift them slowly a few times before putting them away.
- **Vacuuming or sweeping:** Keep your knees slightly bent and move with purpose — this counts as weight-bearing movement.
- **Making the bed:** Try lunging one leg forward as you pull up the sheets. It strengthens thighs and improves balance.
- **Stairs:** Take stairs instead of ramps or elevators when safe — going up builds bone, going down challenges balance.

Evening Routine

- **During commercial breaks or between shows:**
  - March in place.
  - Do gentle chair squats.
  - Practice sit-to-stands without using your hands.
- **Before bed:**
  - Do gentle ankle circles and toe taps while sitting on the edge of the bed.

- Stand tall against a wall for 1 minute, shoulders back — great for posture and spine alignment.

Weekend or Outdoor Habits

- **Grocery shopping:** Use reusable bags and carry one in each hand to balance weight evenly.
- **Walking the dog:** Add short hills or uneven ground (if safe) to challenge balance and bone strength.
- **Gardening:** Squat instead of bending at the waist; lifting soil or tools adds resistance naturally.
- **Social time:** Dance, walk with friends, or play light sports — fun movement counts too!

Safety Tips

- Always move slowly and use support if you're unsure of your balance.
- Avoid twisting or jerking motions.
- Make sure floors are clear of clutter to prevent falls.
- Stop if you feel dizzy, unsteady, or short of breath.

The Takeaway

Every movement counts.
The more often you stand, stretch, lift, and move with purpose, the more signals you send your bones to stay strong.
Think of daily tasks as built-in bone builders — not chores, but opportunities for strength.

Section 3

Prepare for Your First Bone Health Visit

Before Your Bone Health Visit

Why It Helps to Prepare

A visit for bone health is different from a regular check-up.
Your medical provider will look at your whole health picture — your past, your lifestyle, your medications, and sometimes even your family history — to understand why your bones might be weaker and how to make them stronger.

The more information you bring, the more accurate and helpful your care will be.
Think of this as your "bone health homework" — getting organized before your visit helps your provider give you the best advice and treatment plan.

Bring these items or details to your appointment. It's okay to write them down if it's easier to remember:

What to Bring	Why It Matters
Your medication and supplement bottles	Your provider needs to see exact doses, brands, and ingredients. Some vitamins or prescriptions can affect bones or interfere with each other.
Any previous bone density scan reports (DEXA)	This helps your provider see if your bone strength has changed over time.
Recent lab results	Blood work like calcium, vitamin D, thyroid, or hormone levels can help find the cause of bone loss.
List of fractures or broken bones	Include how each break happened. A break from a simple fall may suggest fragile bones.

Family history	If your parents or siblings had hip fractures or osteoporosis, your risk is higher.
Medical history	Note any major illnesses (thyroid disease, kidney disease, cancer, rheumatoid arthritis, digestive disorders, or surgeries like hysterectomy or gastric bypass).
Gynecologic history (for women)	Include the age you started menopause and any use of hormone therapy or birth control that affected hormones.
Cancer treatment history	Radiation, chemotherapy, or hormone-blocking medications can affect bone density and medication choices.
Lifestyle notes	Write down how active you are, what your diet is like, and if you use alcohol, tobacco, or caffeine regularly.
List of recent falls or balance problems	These are key clues for fall prevention planning.

Questions Your Provider May Ask You

1. Have you ever had a bone density scan (DEXA)? When and where? ____

2. Have you ever broken a bone as an adult? ____

3. What medicines, vitamins, or supplements do you take every day? ____

4. Have you used steroids (like prednisone) for more than a few months? ____

5. Do you smoke, or have you smoked in the past? ____

6. How much alcohol do you drink in a week? ____

7. How much dairy or calcium do you get in your diet? ____

8. Do you take a vitamin D supplement? ____

9. How much sunlight do you get? ____

10. What kind of exercise do you do, and how often? ____________

____

11. For women: At what age did menopause begin? Did you ever take hormone therapy? ____________

____

12. For men: Have you ever had low testosterone? ____________

____

13. Does anyone in your family have osteoporosis or a history of hip fracture? ____________

____

14. Have you noticed any change in your height, posture, or back pain? ____________

____

Questions You May Want to Ask Your Provider

Bringing your own list of questions helps you feel confident and ensures you leave with answers.
Here are some good examples to start with:

1. When should I have a bone density test?

2. Do I need any blood work to check for causes of bone loss?

3. Am I at risk for secondary osteoporosis?

4. What lifestyle changes would help my bones the most?

5. Should I take calcium or vitamin D supplements? How much?

6. What kind of exercise is best for me?

7. Are there medications that can help build or protect my bones?

8. How often will I need checkups or follow-up scans?

Your Bone Health Visit Checklist

☐ Medication and supplement bottles (or a detailed list)
☐ Bone density (DEXA) results, if you have them
☐ Recent blood work
☐ List of past fractures or broken bones
☐ Family history of bone loss or fractures
☐ Medical and surgical history (especially hormone or cancer-related)
☐ Notes about lifestyle (diet, exercise, smoking, alcohol use)
☐ History of falls or balance concerns
☐ Written list of questions for your provider

Tip: If you can, bring a family member or friend to help take notes during your appointment. Two sets of ears are better than one!

The Takeaway

Preparing before your appointment helps your provider see the full picture — not just your bones, but your overall health.
That preparation means fewer surprises, clearer answers, and a care plan that truly fits you.

Section 4

Why Osteoporosis Matters

How to use this book

The Silent Problem

- Osteoporosis often develops quietly.
- You can't feel your bones getting weaker, and most people don't know they have it until a bone breaks. By that time, bone strength may already be very low.
- That's why it's called the **"silent disease."**
- But the good news is — bone loss can be found *before* a break happens. That's the goal of screening, lab work, and preventive care.

Why Fracture Prevention Matters

A fracture is more than a broken bone—it can change your daily life.

For older adults, even a small fall may mean:

- **Pain and long recovery** that can last months
- **Loss of independence** with walking or driving
- **Medical complications** such as blood clots, infection, or pneumonia
- **Fear of falling again,** which often leads to moving less—and losing even more bone and muscle

---

Type of Fracture	What Happens	Why It Matters
Wrist	Fall onto an outstretched hand	Often the first sign of weak bones; may limit grip strength
Spine (Compression)	A vertebra collapses, sometimes from a cough or twist	Causes back pain, height loss, or stooped posture
Hip	Usually from a simple fall	Often requires surgery; one in five adults may die within a year of a hip fracture
Shoulder/ Upper Arm	Fall onto arm or side	Leads to stiffness and limited motion
Foot/Ankle	Missed step or uneven ground	Causes swelling, poor balance, and fear of walking

Break the Cycle, Keep Your Freedom

When bones get weaker, people move less—and then bones get even weaker.
Your move today:

1) Walk 10 minutes
2) Do 10 sit-to-stands from a chair
3) Clear one tripping hazard at home. Small steps done daily protect your bones and your confidence.

1. Wrist Fractures

Usually happens when someone falls and tries to catch themselves with their hand.

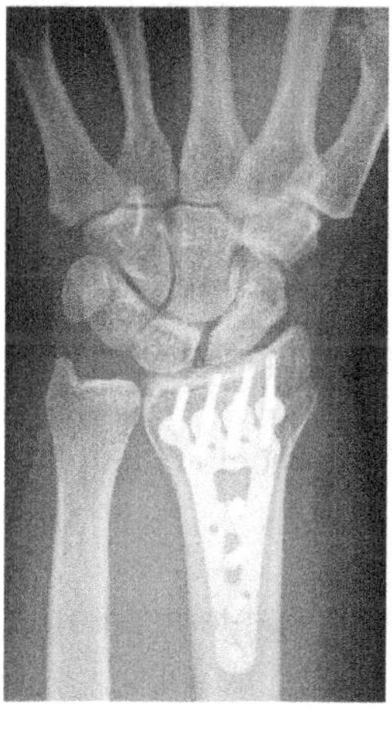

Treatment often includes a cast, or sometimes surgery with a metal plate and screws.

A wrist fracture is often an *early warning sign* of osteoporosis — a signal to check bone density and take steps to protect against future fractures.

2. Spinal Compression Fractures

Occur when one or more spinal bones (vertebrae) collapse slightly. This can happen from a minor fall or even coughing, sneezing, or lifting something light.

Compression fractures can cause a “**domino effect**” — one fracture increases pressure on nearby bones, raising the risk of more spinal fractures.

3. Hip Fractures

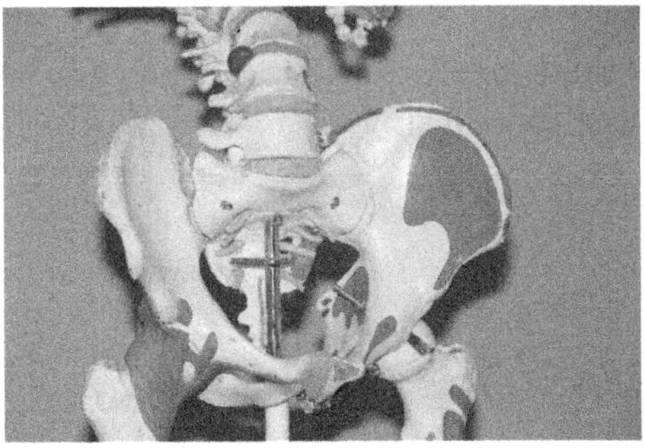

One of the most serious complications of osteoporosis.
Usually caused by a simple fall, especially in older adults, and almost always requires surgery.

- Difficulty walking or climbing stairs — some people may need a cane or walker permanently

- Greater risk of infection, blood clots, or pneumonia during recovery

- Many people lose independence or require long-term care

Why it matters:

- Up to **20–30% of older adults die within one year of a hip fracture**, and about **half lose the ability to live independently.** According to the AAOS and UpToDate.

- That's why hip fracture prevention is one of the most important goals in osteoporosis care.

---

4. Shoulder and Upper Arm Fractures

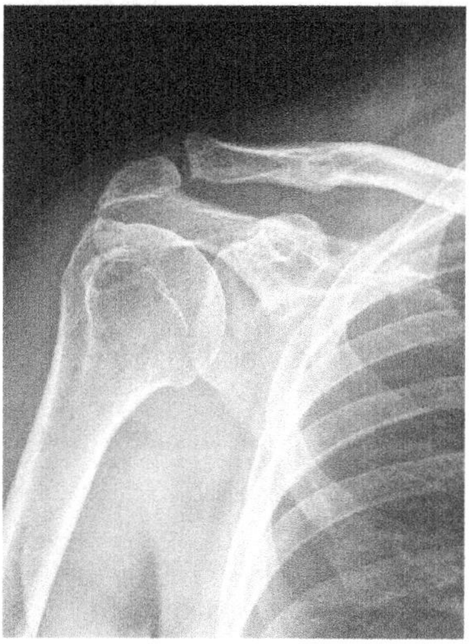

- Can occur from a simple trip or fall, especially landing on an outstretched arm.

- Treatment can include a sling, physical therapy, or surgery (with plates or even shoulder replacement).

5. Foot and Ankle Fractures

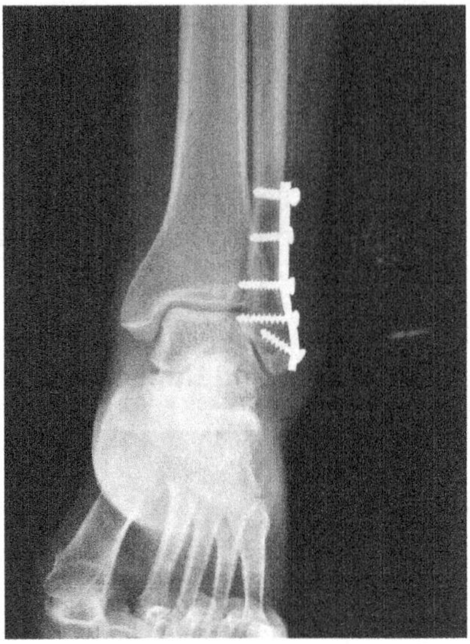

- Common in both men and women with low bone mass.
- May happen from tripping, stepping off a curb, or twisting the ankle.
- Usually treated with a boot or cast, sometimes with surgery if bones are displaced.

Consequences:

- Pain and swelling that can last months
- Reduced ability to walk long distances or stand for long periods
- Balance changes that increase the risk of future falls
- Loss of confidence in walking on uneven ground

Even when healed, ankle and foot fractures can slow mobility and independence, especially if multiple fractures occur over time.

The Big Picture

Osteoporosis care isn't just about X-rays or numbers—it's about staying active, confident, and connected.
Strong bones help you:

- Avoid pain and surgery
- Stay mobile and independent
- Enjoy family, hobbies, and travel
- Move without fear

Every healthy choice—good nutrition, safe movement, regular checkups—helps **preserve your freedom and peace of mind**.

Section 5

Risk Factors for Osteoporosis

You Have More Control Than You Think

You Have More Control Than You Think

- Osteoporosis risk grows with age, hormones, and lifestyle—but most factors can be improved.

- Understanding your risks isn't about blame; it's about empowerment.

---

1. Age and Family History

- **Age**: Everyone loses some bone density as they get older. After age 40, bone breakdown often outpaces rebuilding.

- **Family History**: If your parents or grandparents had osteoporosis or hip fractures, you're more likely to develop it too. Bone density is significantly influenced by genetics (heritability estimated at 60–80 %).

What You Can Do:

- Start bone-friendly habits early — but remember, it's *never too late*.
- Ask your provider when to begin bone density testing (often age 65 for women, 70 for men, or earlier if you have risk factors).

2. Hormonal Changes

- **Women**: After menopause, estrogen levels drop sharply, which accelerates bone loss. In U.S. populations, osteoporosis prevalence in women aged 50+ is about 18.8%. CDC.gov
- **Men**: Low testosterone can also weaken bones. Men aged 50+ have an osteoporosis prevalence of about 4.2%.

What to do: talk with your provider about hormone testing, sleep, stress, and exercise—all of which support healthy levels.

---

3. Medical Conditions & Medications

Thyroid disease, rheumatoid arthritis, diabetes, celiac disease, kidney problems, cancer therapy, long-term steroids, and some stomach or seizure drugs can thin bone.

What to do:

- Never stop taking medication on your own.
- Ask if bone-protective treatment or vitamin D/calcium supplements are needed.
- Keep an updated medication list for every visit.

---

4. Lifestyle Factors You Can Change

- **Smoking** slows bone building—cutting back or quitting helps immediately.
- **Alcohol** beyond one (women) or two (men) drinks daily interferes with calcium balance.
- **Inactivity** weakens bones—aim for 30 minutes of walking, dancing, or light weights most days.
- **Poor diet** reduces bone fuel—focus on dairy or fortified milk, leafy greens, beans, and fish.
- **Falls** cause most fractures—improve balance, clear clutter, and use grab bars where needed.

---

5. Weight, Nutrition & Sleep

- Being underweight reduces bone reserves; being significantly overweight strains joints.
- Aim for a balanced weight, enough protein, fruits, and vegetables, and 7–8 hours of sleep each night.
- Chronic stress and poor rest raise cortisol, which harms bone renewal.

6. Vision & Balance

- Poor eyesight or medications that cause dizziness increase fall risk.

- Get yearly eye exams and ask a physical therapist to check your balance.

---

7. Prevention in Action

Small daily steps add up:

☐ Walk 10 minutes twice a day
☐ Take calcium + vitamin D as directed
☐ Avoid tobacco and limit alcohol
☐ Schedule regular DEXA scans
☐ Keep a safe, well-lit home

The Takeaway

- You can't change your age or family history—but you can change **how your bones age with you.**
- Half of adults over 50 have low bone mass or osteoporosis, yet most fractures are preventable.
- Consistent care—smart diet, movement, medication, and fall safety—keeps you strong, steady, and independent for years to come.

Here's What You Can Start Today:

- ☐ Add a **10-minute walk** to your daily routine.
- ☐ Take your **calcium and vitamin D** as recommended.
- ☐ Quit smoking or cut back on alcohol.
- ☐ Get your **bone density scan** and review results with your provider.
- ☐ Make your home safer to prevent falls.
- ☐ Keep an updated list of your medications and bring it to every appointment.

Section 6

Myth or Fact?
Clearing Up Common Confusion About Osteoporosis

Let's Test What You Know!

🦴 1. Only women get osteoporosis.

Myth!

- While women are more likely to get osteoporosis, **men can get it too.**
- About 1 in 5 men over age 50 will have a fracture caused by weak bones.
- Men with low testosterone, long-term steroid use, or certain medical conditions are especially at risk.

🥛 2. If I drink milk, my bones will always stay strong.

Myth!

- Milk and dairy are good sources of calcium, but that's only part of the story.
- Your bones also need **vitamin D, protein, magnesium, and exercise** to stay strong.
- It's about the *whole lifestyle*, not just one food.

🧍 3. Osteoporosis is just a normal part of getting older.

Myth!

- Bone loss does happen with age — but osteoporosis is **not inevitable.**
- You can protect your bones with good nutrition, exercise, fall prevention, and, if needed, medications.
- Plenty of people stay strong and active well into their 80s and 90s!

🏃 4. Exercise can actually make my bones stronger.

Fact!

- Weight-bearing exercise — like walking, dancing, or light resistance training — helps bones rebuild themselves.
- When muscles pull on bones, it signals the body to make them stronger.
- Just 30 minutes of movement most days can make a big difference.

⚖️ 5. Thin people are less likely to get osteoporosis.

Myth!

- People who are **underweight** have less "bone reserve" and may lose bone faster.
- Being too thin can also mean you're not getting enough nutrients or estrogen to protect bone.
- Aim for a healthy, balanced weight — not too low, not too high.

💊 6. Taking calcium supplements is all I need.

Myth!

- Calcium is important, but your body also needs **vitamin D** to absorb it — and **exercise** to help it work.
- Supplements can help if you don't get enough calcium from food, but they're only part of the plan.

---

7. You can feel it when your bones are getting weaker.

Myth!

- Osteoporosis doesn't cause pain until a fracture happens.
- That's why it's called the "silent disease."
- You may not know you have it unless you get a **bone density test (DEXA).**

8. Drinking alcohol affects my bones.

Fact!

- More than 1–2 drinks a day can make it harder for your body to absorb calcium and increase your fall risk.
- Moderation is key — your bones will thank you!

9. It's too late to do anything about bone loss once it starts.

Myth! (And a big one!)

- It's *never too late.*
- Exercise, calcium, vitamin D, and medications can all slow bone loss and sometimes help rebuild bone.
- People in their 70s, 80s, and even 90s can still make improvements.

10. Osteoporosis only affects bones.

Myth!

- When bones break, it can affect your whole life — your movement, confidence, and independence.
- But preventing fractures helps you stay active, social, and happy.
  Strong bones mean a strong life!

🏆 Your Score Doesn't Matter — Your Knowledge Does!

- If you got something wrong, don't worry — you're not alone!
- Most people have heard at least one of these myths before.
- Now you know the truth: Osteoporosis is preventable, treatable, and manageable at any age.
- You can take charge of your bone health starting today.

Next up:
In the next chapter, we'll learn how bone strength is measured — and how a simple scan can help spot osteoporosis long before a fracture happens.

Section 7

Testing and Diagnosis

How We Measure Bone Strength

Why Testing Matters

- Osteoporosis is often silent — you can't feel your bones getting weaker.
- That's why testing is so important. A bone density test can find problems *early,* before a fracture ever happens.
- It's quick, painless, and gives your provider valuable information about how strong your bones really are.

The DEXA Scan: The Gold Standard

- The most common and reliable test for bone strength is the **DEXA scan**, which stands for **Dual-Energy X-ray Absorptiometry** (say it "deck-suh").
- It uses very low-dose X-rays to measure how dense (or thick) your bones are.

What to Expect:

- You lie on a padded table while the scanner passes over your hips and lower spine.
- It takes about **10–15 minutes**.
- You don't feel anything — it's painless and noninvasive.
- You don't need an IV, dye, or any injections.
- You can stay dressed (just avoid zippers, metal buttons, or jewelry).

The test measures how much calcium and other minerals are packed into your bones. The result shows whether your bones are normal, slightly thin (**osteopenia**), or significantly weak (**osteoporosis**).

Understanding Your DEXA Results

- Your bone density test, called a **DEXA scan**, tells how strong your bones are compared to others.
- Think of it like a **bone strength scorecard.**
- It helps your provider see if your bones are solid, thinning, or fragile.

Your Report Has Two Numbers:

Result Type	What It Compares	What It Means
T-score	Your bone density compared to a healthy 30-year-old adult	Used to diagnose osteopenia or osteoporosis
Z-score	Your bone density compared to others your same age, sex, and size	Helps find unusual causes of bone loss

---

A Simple Way to Understand the T-Score

Think of your **T-score** like a **grading scale** for your bones:

- **0** is a "perfect score" — strong, healthy bone (like getting an A).
- **-1.0 to -2.5** is like getting a B–C — your bone is a bit thinner than average (called *osteopenia*).
- **Below -2.5** is like getting a D–F — your bone is fragile and in the *osteoporosis* range.
- So, the **lower (more negative) the number**, the thinner and weaker the bone.
- You can think of it as how far below "average strength" your bones are.

Another Way to Picture It

- Imagine your bones are a **wall made of bricks.**
- A healthy 30-year-old has a wall with all the bricks tightly in place.
- Each step down (from 0 to -1, to -2.5, etc.) means a few bricks are missing or worn down.
- If enough bricks are gone, the wall becomes unstable — that's osteoporosis.
- The DEXA scan tells us how solid your "brick wall" still is.

Z-Score (Bonus Information)

- Your **Z-score** compares you to people your same age and body type.
- If your Z-score is much lower than expected, your provider might look for a medical reason (like thyroid or vitamin D problems).
- Think of it as checking if your bones are unusually thin for *you*, not just for your age group.

How Often Should You Get Tested?

Testing frequency depends on your age, gender, and risk factors.

In the United States (National Osteoporosis Foundation NOF & Endocrine Society recommend):

- **Women age 65+** and **men age 70+**: should have a DEXA scan.
- **Postmenopausal women or men 50–69 with risk factors** (like a fracture, steroid use, or early menopause): should test earlier.
- **Repeat testing:** every **1–2 years**, or sooner if you start a bone medication or have a new fracture.

Always ask your healthcare provider how often your test should be repeated — some people need it more or less often depending on their bone health plan.

The Takeaway

- Your DEXA scan is your **bone health report card.**
- It doesn't just tell you where you are — it helps track how your bones respond to treatment and lifestyle changes.
- The goal is to keep your numbers stable — or even move them back toward "normal."

New and Emerging Bone Density Tools

While DEXA remains the gold standard, new technologies are being studied to make bone testing even easier.

1. **REMS** (Radiofrequency Echographic Multi Spectrometry)

- A new **ultrasound-based** test that measures bone density and bone quality without radiation.

- It can be done at the heel, spine, or hip in just a few minutes.

- It's showing promise in research for being portable and highly accurate.

- However, it's **not yet widely available** in the U.S. and is still being studied for how well it predicts fracture risk compared to DEXA.

Bottom line: REMS may become more common in the future, but for now, DEXA is still the main test used worldwide.

2. **Quantitative CT** (QCT)

- A special type of CT scan that can measure bone density in 3D.

- It's more detailed but uses higher radiation, so it's usually reserved for research or special cases.

3. **FRAX Score**

- Even without imaging, your provider can estimate your fracture risk using the **FRAX tool** — a questionnaire developed by the World Health Organization.

It calculates your 10-year chance of breaking a bone based on:

- Age and sex
- Weight and height
- Prior fractures
- Smoking or alcohol use
- Family history
- Corticosteroid or hormone use
- Bone density (if available)

You can even try it yourself at:
https://www.fraxplus.org/calculation-tool

Preparing for a DEXA Scan

- You can eat normally before the test.
- Don't take **calcium supplements** for 24 hours before your scan (it can affect accuracy).
- Avoid wearing clothes with metal fasteners.
- Tell your provider if you've recently had a CT scan or contrast study.

Questions to Ask Your Provider

1. When should I get my first or next bone density scan?
2. What do my results mean for my risk of fracture?
3. Has my bone density changed since my last test?
4. What can I do to improve my numbers?
5. When will we recheck?

The Takeaway

- A DEXA scan doesn't just measure numbers — it measures *opportunity.*
- Every scan is a chance to spot problems early and take action before a fracture happens.
- The technology may change over time, but one thing stays the same: the sooner you know your bone health, the sooner you can start protecting it.

Section 8

Lab Tests and Secondary Causes

What Your Blood Can Tell Us About Your Bones

Why Lab Tests Matter

- Bone health isn't just about bone density.
- Sometimes, bones weaken because of **another hidden problem** — such as a hormone imbalance, vitamin deficiency, or medication side effect.
- That's why your provider may order blood and urine tests to look for "secondary causes" of osteoporosis.
- These tests help find the *why* behind bone loss, so your treatment can be personalized.
- Most of these are **simple blood draws** — no fasting, no special preparation, and no pain beyond a small pinch.

Common Blood Tests for Bone Health

Below is a list of common tests, what their names mean, and what they help your provider understand.

1. **CBC** – Complete Blood Count

What it means: Measures your red blood cells, white blood cells, and platelets.
Why it matters: Low red cells (**anemia**) can make you tired and sometimes signal hidden bleeding or illness.

- Unusual results may suggest conditions that affect bone marrow or overall health.

---

2. **CMP** – Comprehensive Metabolic Panel

What it means: A group of tests that check your kidney, liver, and electrolyte balance.
Why it matters: Your **kidneys** help control calcium and vitamin D balance. Your **liver** activates vitamin D.

- Abnormal results can explain why bones aren't rebuilding properly.

(Sometimes your provider may order a "BMP" — Basic Metabolic Panel — which is a shorter version that checks fewer things.)

---

3. **Calcium** (Total and Ionized)

What it means: Measures the main mineral that makes bones hard and strong.

- **Total calcium** looks at the overall level in your blood.
- **Ionized calcium** measures the "active" form your body actually uses.

Why it matters: If calcium is too low or too high, it could mean a hormone problem or a vitamin D issue.

---

4. **Phosphorus**

What it means: Another mineral that works hand-in-hand with calcium.

Why it matters: Phosphorus helps form bone structure.
Too much or too little can be a clue to kidney disease, hormone imbalance, or poor nutrition.

5. **Magnesium**

What it means: A mineral that helps your body use calcium and vitamin D.

Why it matters: Low magnesium can weaken bones and interfere with bone rebuilding.

---

6. **PTH** – Parathyroid Hormone

What it means: A hormone made by the **parathyroid glands** (tiny glands behind your thyroid).

Why it matters: PTH keeps calcium levels in balance.

- When calcium is low, PTH rises to pull calcium out of your bones.
- When calcium is high, PTH should drop.
  Abnormal levels can cause bone thinning over time.

---

7. **Thyroid Tests** – TSH and Free T4

What it means:

- **TSH (Thyroid Stimulating Hormone):** Tells your thyroid how active to be.
- **Free T4 (Thyroxine):** Measures the actual thyroid hormone circulating in your blood.

Why it matters: If your thyroid is **overactive** (hyperthyroidism) or your thyroid medication dose is too high, bones can lose calcium too quickly.

---

8. **Vitamin D** (25-hydroxy Vitamin D)

What it means: The best test for checking your vitamin D level.

Why it matters: Vitamin D helps your body absorb calcium from food and supplements. Low levels are one of the most common causes of bone loss.

Normal Range: Often 30–100 ng/mL (your lab report will list exact values).

---

9. **Sex Hormones**

For Women: Estrogen (Estradiol) and **FSH (Follicle Stimulating Hormone)** may be checked to see if menopause or low hormones are affecting bone loss.

For Men: Testosterone may be tested if bone loss seems rapid or unexplained. Low testosterone is a major but often overlooked cause of osteoporosis in men.

---

10. **CTX or NTX** – Bone Turnover Markers

What it means: CTX (C-terminal telopeptide) and NTX (N-terminal telopeptide) measure small fragments released when bone breaks down.

Why it matters: High levels mean your bones are breaking down faster than they're rebuilding. These tests help providers track how well medications are working over time.

---

11. **Celiac Screening** (TTG or EMA Antibodies)

What it means: Looks for celiac disease, which causes your body to react to gluten.

Why it matters: Celiac disease can make it hard to absorb calcium, vitamin D, and other nutrients — leading to bone loss.

---

12. **SPEP and UPEP** – Protein Tests

What it means: (Serum Protein Electrophoresis) and UPEP (Urine Protein Electrophoresis) check for abnormal proteins made by the bone marrow.

Why it matters: These tests look for rare causes of bone weakness such as multiple myeloma — a cancer that affects bone strength.

Optional or Additional Tests

Your provider may order other tests based on your situation:

- **Cortisol levels** – to check for Cushing's disease (too much steroid hormone)

- **Kidney function tests** – if you take long-term medications or have chronic illness (simple ones are included in the BMP/CMP

- **24-hour urine calcium** – to measure how much calcium you lose in your urine

---

How These Tests Are Done

- Almost all are **simple blood draws.**

- A few may use a **urine sample.**

- Most don't require fasting.

Results usually return within a few days.

What Happens Next

Your provider will look at all the pieces together — blood tests, bone scan, and your medical history — to find patterns and possible causes.
If an underlying problem is found (like low vitamin D or thyroid issues), treating it can often **improve your bone health naturally.**

All in Plain Language

Test	Checks For	Why It Helps
CBC	Blood cell counts	Finds anemia or bone marrow issues
CMP	Kidney & liver function	Looks for causes of calcium or vitamin D imbalance
Calcium	Bone mineral levels	Identifies calcium deficiency or excess
Phosphorus	Mineral balance	Works with calcium to build bone
Magnesium	Mineral that activates vitamin D	Helps with calcium absorption
PTH	Parathyroid hormone	Detects overactive glands pulling calcium from bone
Thyroid (TSH, T4)	Thyroid activity	Finds overactive metabolism causing bone loss
Vitamin D	Vitamin for calcium absorption	Checks if you're getting enough sunlight or supplements
CTX / NTX	Bone breakdown markers	Shows how fast your bones are turning over
Estrogen / Testosterone	Sex hormones	Detects menopause or low testosterone effects
Celiac screening	Gluten intolerance	Finds poor nutrient absorption
SPEP / UPEP	Protein balance	Screens for rare bone marrow conditions

The Takeaway

- Lab tests tell your bone story — from the nutrients you absorb to the hormones that keep bones strong.
- They don't just look for disease — they help your provider personalize your plan for stronger, healthier bones.

Section 9

Medications for Osteoporosis

Understanding Your Treatment Options

Why Medications Matter

If your bones are already weak, healthy habits alone may not be enough to make them strong again. That's where **medications** can help.

Osteoporosis medicines work by doing one or both of these things:

- **Slow down bone loss** (so you stop losing calcium too fast)
- **Help your body build new bone**

Your medical provider will choose what's right for you based on your **bone density**, **fracture history**, **age**, and **other health conditions**.

---

1. Bisphosphonates – "Bone Protectors" *(They slow down bone loss.)*

Generic Name	Brand Name(s)	How You Take It
Alendronate	Fosamax®, Binosto®	Pill – once a week
Risedronate	Actonel®, Atelvia®	Pill – weekly or monthly
Ibandronate	Boniva®	Pill (monthly) or IV every 3 months
Zoledronic acid	Reclast®, Zometa®	IV infusion once a year

How They Work:

- These medicines help your bones "hold on" to calcium and stay dense.
- They slow the cells that break down bone, giving your body time to rebuild.

Who They Help:

- Women and men with osteoporosis or bone thinning (osteopenia)
- People taking long-term steroids like prednisone
- Those at risk for fractures

Tips for Taking Pills:

- Take in the **morning with a full glass of water** before eating or drinking.
- Stay **upright for 30–60 minutes** afterward to protect your stomach.
- If pills upset your stomach, ask about **IV forms** (Reclast® or Boniva®).
- After **3–5 years**, your provider may give you a "break" if your bones are stable.

---

2. Denosumab – “The Antibody Shot” *(Slows down bone loss, like a pause button.)*

Generic Name	Brand Name(s)	How You Take It
Denosumab	Prolia® (for osteoporosis), Xgeva® (for cancer-related bone loss)	Injection every 6 months

How It Works: It blocks a signal that tells your body to break down bone. Think of it like hitting the *pause* button on bone loss.

Who It Helps:

- People who can't take bisphosphonates
- Those with **kidney problems**
- Postmenopausal women and men with a high fracture risk

Tips:

- Must be given **every 6 months on time** — missing doses can cause fast bone loss.
- You'll likely take **calcium and vitamin D** with it.
- **Don't stop suddenly** — bone loss can rebound quickly.

---

3. Anabolic Medications – "Bone Builders" *(They help your body make new bone.)*

Generic Name	Brand Name(s)	How You Take It
Teriparatide	Forteo®	Daily injection (at home)
Abaloparatide	Tymlos®	Daily injection (at home)
Romosozumab	Evenity®	Monthly injections at your doctor's office for 12 months

How They Work: These are "bone-building boosters." They help your body form **new, stronger bone** instead of just slowing bone loss.

Who They Help:

- People with **severe osteoporosis** or **multiple fractures**
- Those whose bones didn't improve on other medicines
- Patients with **very low T-scores (–3.0 or lower)**

Tips:

- Usually used for **12–24 months**, then followed by another medicine (like Reclast® or Prolia®) to keep the new bone strong.
- You'll have **regular blood tests** to check calcium levels.
- Not used in people with **bone cancer, Paget's disease**, or **high calcium levels**.

4. Hormone-Related Therapies *(Helpful for some women after menopause.)*

A. Estrogen Therapy

- Estrogen helps protect bones, but levels drop after menopause.
- Hormone therapy can slow bone loss in women early after menopause.

Common Brands: Premarin®, Estrace®, Climara®, Vivelle-Dot®

How It's Taken: Pill, patch, or cream

Important Notes:

- Works best when started **near menopause**, not many years later.
- Not for women with a history of **breast cancer, stroke, or blood clots.**
- Always discuss risks and benefits with your medical provider.

B. SERMs – "Estrogen Helpers" (selective estrogen receptor modulator–*These act like estrogen in bones but not in other parts of the body.)*

Generic Name	Brand Name(s)	How You Take It
Raloxifene	Evista®	Daily pill

How It Works: Acts like estrogen in the bones to **prevent bone loss** without affecting the breast or uterus.

Who It Helps:

- Postmenopausal women who can't take estrogen therapy.

Notes:

- May increase the risk of **leg blood clots**, so not for people with a history of clotting.

---

5. Calcitonin – "The Nose Spray Option"

Generic Name	Brand Name(s)	How You Take It
Calcitonin-salmon	Miacalcin®, Fortical®	Nasal spray or injection

How It Works:

- Calcitonin is a natural hormone that helps control calcium.
- It slows bone loss and may reduce **spine fracture pain**.

Who It Helps:

- People who can't take other treatments
- Those needing short-term relief from **spinal fracture pain**

Why So Many Choices?

Different medicines help in different ways — your provider will match them to what your bones need most.

If You Need To...	Medication Type
Slow bone loss	Bisphosphonates, Denosumab, SERMs, Calcitonin
Build new bone	Forteo®, Tymlos®, Evenity®
Manage menopause-related bone loss	Estrogen or Raloxifene (Evista®)
Ease spine fracture pain	Calcitonin (Miacalcin®, Fortical®)

The Takeaway

- There's no one-size-fits-all treatment for osteoporosis.
- Some medicines stop bone loss; others build new bone.
- The best plan is the one that fits *your* health, *your* lifestyle, and *your* comfort.
- Always ask questions and stay involved — your bones will thank you.

Medication Management & Safety

How to Take Your Bone Medicine the Right Way

- Osteoporosis medicines work best when you know how to take them safely and consistently.
- Missing doses or combining them with the wrong pills can make them less effective.

Stay on Schedule

- Daily or Weekly Pills (Fosamax®, Actonel®) — Take first thing in the morning with a full glass of water. Stay upright for at least 30 minutes before eating or drinking anything else.
- Monthly Pills (Boniva®) — Mark your calendar so you don't forget the date.
- Shots or Infusions (Prolia®, Reclast®) — Put reminders in your phone or ask your clinic to schedule the next dose before you leave.
- Review these recommendations with your provider, but typically If you miss a pill → take it the next morning; if you miss a shot → call your provider. Never double up.

Check Your Other Medications

Some medicines can keep calcium or bone pills from working right:

- Heartburn meds (omeprazole, pantoprazole) — may lower calcium absorption.
- Thyroid replacement (levothyroxine) — takes at least 4 hours apart from calcium or iron.
- Water pills (loop diuretics) — can increase calcium loss.
- Long-term steroids (prednisone) — ask about extra bone protection.

Bring every medication and supplement bottle to each visit so your provider can double-check interactions. You can also consider talking to your Pharmacist about possible interactions.

When to Call Your Provider

- New or unusual thigh, groin, or jaw pain
- Swallowing trouble or chest burning after a pill
- Muscle cramps, tingling, or weakness
- Missed an injection or infusion appointment

Your care team wants to know early — it's much easier to adjust treatment than to fix a broken bone later.

Common Questions

Q: Why do some medications help with "low calcium" while others don't?

- Because some medicines **move calcium back into the bones**, while others help **your body use calcium better.**

For example:

- Bisphosphonates and denosumab help bones **keep** calcium instead of losing it.
- Anabolic medicines help **add** new calcium to bones by stimulating growth.
- If your calcium or vitamin D is too low, your provider may fix that before starting any bone medication.

Q: Can I take more than one medication?

- Usually not at the same time.
- However, you may switch from one to another or follow an "anabolic first, antiresorptive second" plan — building bone first, then maintaining it.

Q: How long will I need treatment?

- Most people take osteoporosis medication for **3–5 years**, sometimes longer.
- Your provider will review your bone density scans and labs to decide when (or if) you can take a break.

Your Role Matters Too

Medications work best when combined with:

- Daily **calcium** and **vitamin D**
- **Exercise** (especially weight-bearing activities)
- **Not smoking** and limiting alcohol
- Regular **bone density testing** to track progress

The Takeaway

- These medications don't just "add minerals" — they help your bones rebuild and protect themselves.
- Knowing the names, how they work, and what to expect helps you feel confident and in control of your care.

Section 10

Nutrition & Bone Health

Feeding Your Bones for Strength and Longevity

Food Is the Foundation of Bone Health

- Your bones are built from the nutrients you eat.
- Every bite you take can either **feed your bones** or leave them hungry for the minerals they need.

The good news?

- You don't need fancy diets or expensive powders — just everyday foods that provide calcium, vitamin D, protein, and other key nutrients.

🥛 **Calcium**: The Building Block of Bone

Why You Need It: Calcium is the main mineral that gives bones their hardness and strength.

If your diet doesn't supply enough calcium, your body will **borrow it from your bones** to keep your heart and muscles working — which leads to bone loss over time.

How Much Calcium Do You Need?

Age / Stage	Daily Calcium Goal
Children (9–18 years)	1,300 mg
Adults (19–50 years)	1,000 mg
Women 51+ & Men 71+	1,200 mg
Pregnant / Breastfeeding	1,000 mg

- It's best to get calcium from food first.
- If you use supplements, spread them out — your body can only absorb about **500 mg at a time.**

Best Food Sources of Calcium

Food	Serving Size	Calcium (mg)
Milk (any type)	1 cup	300
Yogurt	6 oz	250–300
Cheese (cheddar, mozzarella)	1 oz	200
Fortified almond / soy / oat milk	1 cup	250–450
Fortified orange juice	1 cup	300
Canned salmon (with bones)	3 oz	180
Canned sardines (with bones)	3 oz	325
Collard greens (cooked)	1 cup	260
Kale (cooked)	1 cup	180
White beans (cooked)	1 cup	160
Tofu (made with calcium sulfate)	½ cup	250–300
Almonds	1 oz (23 nuts)	75
Chia seeds	2 Tbsp	180
Fortified breakfast cereal	1 cup	100–200

Choosing the Right Calcium Supplement 💊

There are several kinds of calcium on store shelves — here's what they mean:

Type	What It Is	Best For	When to Take
Calcium Carbonate	Contains the highest amount of elemental calcium (about 40%)	People with normal stomach acid	With food (needs acid to absorb)
Calcium Citrate	Easier to absorb, even with low stomach acid	Older adults, people on heartburn meds, or after weight-loss surgery	Anytime, with or without food
Calcium Lactate / Gluconate	Lower calcium content; used in some fortified foods	Mild supplements or sensitive stomachs	With meals
Calcium Phosphate	Good absorption, less constipation	Alternate option if other forms cause stomach upset	With or without food

Tips for Taking Calcium:

- Split doses into **morning and evening** if you need more than 500 mg per day.
- Drink plenty of water — calcium carbonate can sometimes cause constipation.
- Check the label for the amount of **"elemental calcium"** (that's the usable part).
- Pair it with vitamin D for better absorption.

☀ **Vitamin D**: The Key to Absorbing Calcium

Why You Need It: Vitamin D acts like a "gatekeeper," helping your body absorb calcium from food or supplements into your bloodstream — and then move it into your bones.

Without enough vitamin D, even high-calcium diets won't protect your bones.

Types of Vitamin D: There are two main forms:

Type	Also Called	Where It Comes From	Notes
Vitamin D_2 (Ergocalciferol)	"Plant D"	Mushrooms, fortified foods	Works well but doesn't last as long in the body
Vitamin D_3 (Cholecalciferol)	"Animal D"	Sunlight exposure, fish oil, eggs, dairy, fortified milk	Raises blood levels more effectively; most common in supplements

Most experts prefer Vitamin D_3 because it maintains healthy levels longer, especially in adults.

How Much Vitamin D Do You Need?

Age / Stage	Daily Goal (IU)
Adults 19–70	600–800 IU
Adults 71+	800–1,000 IU
Some people need more if levels are low (as guided by your provider)	

Natural Sources:

- Salmon, tuna, sardines
- Egg yolks
- Fortified milk and cereals
- Mushrooms exposed to sunlight
- 10–15 minutes of sunshine a few days per week (arms and face uncovered)

Other Bone-Building Nutrients

Nutrient	Why It Helps	Food Sources
Protein	Builds bone matrix and muscle strength	Lean meat, dairy, eggs, beans
Magnesium	Helps convert vitamin D to its active form	Nuts, seeds, whole grains
Vitamin K	Directs calcium into bones (not arteries)	Leafy greens, broccoli
Phosphorus	Partners with calcium to harden bone	Dairy, meat, beans
Zinc	Supports bone healing	Shellfish, meat, legumes

Calcium in Everyday Meals (No Measuring Needed)

- **Breakfast combo:** 1 cup milk + 6 oz yogurt ≈ **550–600 mg**
- **Quick lunch:** tuna on whole-grain + 1 cup fortified juice ≈ **400–600 mg**
- **Simple dinner:** 1 oz cheese + broccoli + fortified milk ≈ **500–600 mg**
  Tip: Your body uses about **500 mg at a time**. Spread calcium throughout the day.

Supplements: When Food Isn't Enough

If your provider recommends supplements:

- Choose **calcium citrate** if you have stomach problems or take heartburn medicine.
- Choose **calcium carbonate** if you're generally healthy and want the most calcium per pill.
- Take **vitamin D_3** (cholecalciferol) daily, unless you're vegan — then D_2 is fine.
- Combine calcium + vitamin D in one product only if it fits your total daily goals.

Bone-Healthy Meal Ideas

Simple Meals to Feed Your Bones and Muscles

You don't need fancy recipes — just smart pairings of calcium, vitamin D, protein, and colorful produce.

Meal	Example	Bone Boost Why It Helps
Break fast	Oatmeal made with fortified milk + chia seeds + berries	Calcium + magnesium for strong bone matrix
Lunch	Tuna or salmon salad on whole-grain toast + spinach side	Vitamin D and omega-3s for bone repair
Snack	Yogurt + handful of almonds or walnuts	Protein and healthy fat for healing
Dinner	Grilled chicken + broccoli + sweet potato + glass of fortified milk	Balanced minerals and antioxidants
Evening	Warm milk with cinnamon or soy milk if lactose-free	Calm sleep and extra calcium

Drink plenty of water, limit soda and salt, and remember that food is medicine for your bones.

Key Tips for Bone-Healthy Nutrition

- Eat **calcium-rich foods** at every meal.
- Include a **source of vitamin D** daily.
- Get enough **protein** to maintain muscle and support healing.
- Avoid **excess salt, caffeine, and soda**, which can cause calcium loss.
- Stay **hydrated** — dehydration makes bones and joints more fragile.

The Takeaway

- The best "medicine" for your bones is what you put on your plate.

- Real food, regular sunlight, and smart supplements give your bones everything they need to stay strong for life.

Bone Health for Every Body

- **Lactose-free?** Use fortified soy, almond, or oat milk and leafy greens.

- **Limited sun or darker skin?** Ask about checking **vitamin D**—you may need more.

- **Tight budget?** Canned salmon/sardines (with bones), beans, eggs, and greens are **low-cost** bone foods.

- **Cultural foods count.** Tortillas made with calcium-fortified masa, tofu set with calcium, and leafy greens in stews all help.

🥦 3-Day Bone-Healthy Meal Plan

Simple, Affordable, and Realistic Meals for Stronger Bones

- Healthy eating for bones doesn't have to be complicated or expensive.
- These examples show how to mix calcium, vitamin D, protein, and color into everyday meals.
- Use regular grocery-store foods and adjust portions for your appetite or calorie needs.

Day 1

Meal	Menu	Bone Benefits
Breakfast	Fortified oatmeal with low-fat milk, chia seeds, and sliced banana	Calcium + fiber to start your day strong
Snack	Greek yogurt with almonds	Protein + magnesium for bone structure
Lunch	Grilled salmon salad (spinach, tomatoes, chickpeas, olive oil)	Vitamin D + omega-3s support bone repair
Snack	String cheese or calcium-fortified soy milk	Easy calcium boost
Dinner	Baked chicken breast, roasted broccoli, quinoa, and a small sweet potato	Balanced minerals + protein
Evening	Warm milk or fortified almond milk with cinnamon	Relaxing source of calcium before bed

Day 2

Meal	Menu	Bone Benefits
Breakfast	Scrambled eggs with spinach and whole-grain toast	Vitamin D + iron
Snack	Handful of walnuts or trail mix	Magnesium + healthy fats
Lunch	Turkey and cheese sandwich on whole-grain bread, side of carrot sticks	Protein + vitamin K
Snack	Low-fat yogurt with berries	Calcium + antioxidants
Dinner	Stir-fry with tofu, broccoli, bell peppers, and brown rice	Plant calcium + vitamin C for collagen
Evening	Fortified orange juice or kefir	Vitamin D + probiotics for absorption

---

Day 3

Meal	Menu	Bone Benefits
Breakfast	Smoothie with milk, frozen fruit, spinach, and protein powder	Calcium + vitamin C + protein
Snack	Whole-grain crackers with peanut butter	Protein + magnesium
Lunch	Lentil soup with whole-grain roll and side salad	Fiber + iron + plant protein
Snack	Cottage cheese with pineapple	Calcium + digestive enzymes
Dinner	Baked cod, sautéed kale, and mashed cauliflower	Vitamin D + vitamin K + calcium
Evening	Herbal tea + small square of dark chocolate (70%)	Magnesium + stress relief

Tips:

- Drink water throughout the day — hydration keeps joints cushioned.
- Swap fish, beans, or chicken freely — variety matters more than perfection.
- If lactose-intolerant, use fortified plant milks and leafy greens for calcium.

The goal isn't a "perfect diet." It's steady, balanced choices that feed your bones every day.

For an online source or to consider some personalized meal plans by a registered dietitian, see: https://www.simplehealthoptions.com/

Section 11

Exercise & Physical Therapy for Strong Bones

Move It or Lose It — Why Motion Builds Strength

Why Exercise Is So Important

- Your bones are living tissue — they respond to stress and movement.
- Every time your muscles pull on your bones, it signals your body to build more bone.
- That's why exercise is one of the most powerful tools for preventing and treating osteoporosis.
- Even better: Exercise also improves **balance**, **coordination**, and **muscle strength**, which helps prevent falls — one of the biggest causes of fractures.
- The best part? It's *never too late* to start moving.
- You don't have to run marathons — just find safe, regular movement that fits your body.

🦴 Types of Exercise for Bone Health

There are three main kinds of exercises that help your bones in different ways:

1. **Weight-Bearing Exercise** (for Bone Strength)

- These are activities where your **feet and legs support your body weight** while moving against gravity.
- This kind of movement gently stresses your bones — and they respond by getting denser and stronger.

Why It Matters:

- Bones, especially in your hips, legs, and spine, stay stronger when they "feel" your body weight moving through them.
- Water exercise and biking are great for the heart — but they're *not* weight-bearing, because the water or bike supports your weight for you.

- **Tip:** If walking is your main activity, try adding short bursts of speed or small uphill sections — this adds a healthy challenge for your bones.

---

2. **Resistance or Strength Training** (for Muscle and Bone)

Resistance training uses weights, bands, or even your own body weight to **build muscle strength**, which in turn supports and protects your bones.

Why It Matters:

- Strong muscles act like armor for your bones. They help you stay upright, protect joints, and prevent falls.
- Research shows strength training can increase bone density in the hips and spine, even in older adults.

How Often:

- Aim for **2–3 days per week**.
- Focus on all major muscle groups — arms, legs, back, and core.
- Rest at least one day between strength sessions.
- **Safety Tip:** Start light and build up slowly. A physical therapist can show you how to lift correctly to avoid strain.

Three Spine-Safe Rules (Easy to Remember)

1. No bending and twisting together.
2. Keep things close to your body when lifting.
3. Hips back, chest up when getting out of a chair or picking up items. If an exercise bends or twists your back hard, skip it and ask your PT for a safer version.

3. **Stretching & Flexibility** (for Posture and Safety)

Stretching doesn't directly build bone — but it keeps your muscles and joints flexible, helps you stand taller, and makes movement safer.

Why It Matters:

- Good flexibility improves balance and posture, lowering your risk of falling or twisting awkwardly.
- Tight muscles can pull unevenly on bones and joints, increasing pain or stiffness.
- **Tip:** Avoid forward-bending stretches that round your spine (like touching your toes while standing) if you have spinal osteoporosis — it increases fracture risk.

The Best Routine Combines All Three

A well-balanced bone-health plan should include:

Type	Goal	How Often
Weight-Bearing	Build bone strength	30 min most days, Walking, dancing, stair climbing, low-impact aerobics, light jogging
Resistance / Strength	Build muscle to support bone	2–3 times per week, Hand weights, resistance bands, wall push-ups, sit-to-stands
Stretching / Balance	Improve posture and prevent falls	Daily or at least 3–4 times per week, Yoga, tai chi, gentle daily stretching

- **Start small:** Even 10 minutes twice a day counts.

- The goal is consistency — not perfection.

Exercises to Avoid if You Have Osteoporosis

Some movements can increase fracture risk, especially in the spine:

- Deep forward bends or sit-ups
- Twisting from the waist while carrying weight
- Jumping or running on hard surfaces if you have balance issues
- Heavy overhead lifting without support
- Sudden jerky movements

A physical therapist can show you safe alternatives for each of these.

When to See a Physical Therapist

A **physical therapist (PT)** trained in bone health can:

- Design a safe, personalized program based on your bone density and fitness level

- Teach proper form to avoid injury

- Show how to improve balance and reduce fall risk

- Help you manage posture and pain after fractures

Ask your provider for a referral to a PT who specializes in osteoporosis or senior fitness.

Hospital-based Osteoporosis & Exercise Resources

1. **Duke Health — Osteoporosis Clinic & Physical Therapy**
   Duke's Osteoporosis program mentions that their **physical therapists teach strength training, balance exercises, posture, flexibility** to prevent falls and fractures. https://www.dukehealth.org/treatments/endocrinology/osteoporosis. This is a strong example of an academic medical center integrating exercise into bone health care.

2. **Harvard Health – "Exercises for Bone Strength"**
   Harvard Health publishes a guide with **seven workouts and 60 exercises** specifically designed to improve bone strength. https://www.health.harvard.edu/womens-health/exercises-for-bone-strength
   They also offer background education about why these exercises help.

3. **NIAMS (National Institute of Arthritis and Musculoskeletal and Skin Diseases)**
   NIAMS is a U.S. federal institute and has a patient-facing page titled *"Exercise for Your Bone Health"* that outlines **best types of exercise (weight-bearing, resistance, balance)** for bone health.
   Because it's a federal government source, it's considered credible and non-commercial.

4. **Harvard Health – "Effective Exercises for Osteoporosis"**
   Harvard publishes articles about **effective, safe exercises** for those with or at risk for osteoporosis. https://www.health.harvard.edu/newsletter_article/effective-exercises-for-osteoporosis. Their style is patient-oriented, making it a useful reference to include in your trusted resource list.

5. **BoneHealth & Osteoporosis Foundation (U.S.) + Partner links**
   While not a hospital, the **BoneHealth & Osteoporosis Foundation (formerly NOF)** is a major national nonprofit that provides exercise guides, "Be Bone Strong®" handouts, and safety tips. (Already on your list)
   But additionally, many of their listed **hospital partners and clinical centers** (some academic) provide exercise programs and allied health services — ideal for patients to look locally.

🌟**The Takeaway**

- Bones love movement — but not all movement builds them.
- Weight-bearing and resistance exercise make bones stronger.
- Stretching keeps you flexible, balanced, and confident.
- The secret is to **move safely, move often, and move with purpose.**
- Strong bones are built one step — or one stretch — at a time.

Section 12

Fall Prevention & Home Safety

Protecting Your Bones Starts at Home

Why Fall Prevention Matters

- Most fractures in people with osteoporosis happen after a simple fall — often from standing height or less.
- Falls can lead to broken hips, wrists, or spine fractures, which can seriously affect independence.

The good news?

Most falls are preventable.

- By making small changes to your home, daily habits, and footwear, you can dramatically reduce your risk.

10-Minute Home Tune-Up (Do It Today)

Grab a trash bag and timer. In 10 minutes:
☐ Pick up loose cords and clutter from 1 hallway
☐ Tape down 1 loose rug or remove it
☐ Add 1 night-light from bed to bathroom
☐ Move daily dishes to the **waist-high** shelf
☐ Put non-slip mats in the tub and at the sink

Simple changes prevent **most** home falls

---

1. Strength, Balance, and Awareness

Your first line of defense against falls is your own body.

Tips from Physical Therapists (PTs):

- **Practice balance:** Try standing on one leg while brushing your teeth, or do gentle heel-to-toe walks down a hallway.

- **Build muscle:** Strong legs and core muscles keep you steady.
- **Use support when needed:** There's no shame in using a cane or walker — they protect your bones.
- **Get your vision checked yearly.** Even small changes in eyesight can affect depth perception.
- **Review your medications** with your medical provider or pharmacist. Some may cause dizziness, fatigue, or low blood pressure.

2. Make Your Home Safer

- Occupational therapists specialize in **adapting environments** so you can live independently and safely.
- Here's how they suggest setting up your home room by room:

Entrance and Hallways

- ☐ Keep walkways clear of shoes, cords, and clutter.
- ☐ Use **nonslip mats** at the doorway.
- ☐ Install **motion-sensor lights** or keep a small nightlight near paths used at night.
- ☐ Consider a **ramp** or sturdy **handrails** on both sides of steps

Living Areas

- ☐ Remove **throw rugs** or secure them with double-sided tape or rubber grips.
- ☐ Arrange furniture to create **wide, clear pathways.**
- ☐ Keep items you use daily within easy reach to avoid climbing or bending.

- ☐ If you have pets, train them not to run underfoot or add small bells to collars.

Bathroom

- ☐ Place **grab bars** next to the toilet and inside the shower or tub.
- ☐ Use a **nonslip bathmat** inside and outside the tub.
- ☐ Consider a **shower chair** and a **handheld showerhead.**
- ☐ Keep towels and toiletries within arm's reach — no stretching or twisting.

Bedroom

- ☐ Keep a **lamp or flashlight** by your bed for quick access at night.
- ☐ Avoid slippery floor surfaces — use low-pile rugs with rubber backing.
- ☐ If getting up at night often, consider a **bedside commode** or nearby bathroom nightlight.

Kitchen

- ☐ Store heavy pots and dishes **on lower shelves** to prevent reaching overhead.
- ☐ Use a **sturdy step stool with handholds** — never a chair — if you need to reach high shelves.
- ☐ Keep floors dry and clean up spills right away.
- ☐ Place a **rubber mat** near the sink for stability.

Stairs

- ☐ Add **handrails on both sides.**
- ☐ Keep stairs **well lit** from top to bottom.
- ☐ Apply **nonslip treads** or reflective strips.
- ☐ Don't rush — take your time and carry small loads.

Outdoors

- ☐ Install **good lighting** along walkways and driveways.
- ☐ Keep **paths smooth and free of cracks or moss.**
- ☐ Use **handrails** near steps or porch areas.
- ☐ Wear **supportive shoes** with firm soles and closed heels when gardening or walking.

3. Choose the Right Footwear

Your shoes are your foundation — literally.

Best Options:

- ☐ Closed-toe shoes with **nonslip soles**
- ☐ Low heels (less than 1 inch)
- ☐ Adjustable straps or laces for a secure fit

Avoid:

- ☐ Flip-flops or loose slippers
- ☐ High heels or wedge shoes
- ☐ Socks alone on slick floors

4. Adaptive Tools That Make Life Easier

Occupational therapists often recommend simple tools that help prevent risky bending or stretching:

- Reacher or grabber sticks for picking things up
- Long-handled shoehorns and sponges
- Raised toilet seats or shower benches
- Bedside organizers for medications and glasses
- Nonslip mats and furniture pads for stability

These tools aren't just for older adults — they're smart solutions for anyone who wants to stay independent and safe.

5. Safety Habits That Stick

- ☐ Keep your phone within reach at all times.
- ☐ Tell someone if you've fallen, even if you didn't get hurt — it's a warning sign.
- ☐ Stay hydrated; dehydration can cause dizziness.
- ☐ Move slowly when standing up to avoid light-headedness.
- ☐ Schedule regular checkups for eyes, hearing, and balance.

6. If a Fall Happens

If you do fall:

1. Stay calm and check for pain or injury.
2. Roll onto your side and get to a sturdy surface if you can.
3. If you can't get up safely, call for help or use a medical alert device.

4. Let your provider know — even a small fall can signal balance or medication issues. If hurt, go to the ER, Urgent Care or have an urgent visit with your Primary Provider.

Checklist: Make Your Home Fall-Safe 🏠

☐ Clutter-free floors and hallways
☐ Handrails on all stairs
☐ Grab bars in bathroom
☐ Good lighting throughout home
☐ Nonslip mats in tub and kitchen
☐ Supportive shoes — no slippers or socks only
☐ Step stool with handles (no chairs)
☐ Pet toys and cords kept off walkways
☐ Emergency phone nearby

Recovery After a Fracture

Healing Takes Time — and Patience

- Breaking a bone is never easy, but most people heal well with the right plan.

Recovery usually happens in three phases:

Phase 1: Rest and Protection (Weeks 1–6)

- Follow your provider's instructions about casts, braces, or weight limits.
- Keep moving the rest of your body — gentle ankle circles or arm stretches keep blood flowing.
- Eat plenty of protein, calcium, and vitamin D to fuel healing.

Phase 2: Rebuilding Movement (Weeks 6–12)

- Work with a physical therapist to restore strength and balance.
- Practice safe transfers — rolling to your side before sitting up, using your arms to push up from a chair.
- Add short walks each day as tolerated.

Phase 3: Regaining Confidence (3 months and beyond)

- Resume gentle household tasks and exercise under your provider's guidance.
- Keep fall prevention habits in place.
- Celebrate milestones — each week of steady activity means your bones are getting stronger.

When to call your provider: new pain, swelling, fever, or if you can't bear weight the way you could before.

Healing is not a race — it's a partnership between you, your bones, and your team.

The Takeaway

- You can't prevent every fall, but you can make your home — and your body — much safer.

- Small changes today can protect your bones, your confidence, and your independence tomorrow.

Affiliate Disclosure

Some of the safety and exercise items mentioned in this chapter (such as grab bars, shower chairs, and nonslip mats) may be listed on my Amazon Author Page.
If you purchase through those links, I may earn a small commission at no extra cost to you.
These recommendations are for educational purposes only — always choose what fits your personal safety needs and discuss questions with your healthcare provider or occupational therapist.

Section 13

Osteoporosis in Cancer Survivors and Complex Medical Conditions

Understanding Bone Health When You Have a Medical History

Why Cancer and Chronic Illness Can Affect Bones

- Many people are surprised to learn that cancer treatment or certain long-term medical conditions can affect bone strength.
- The connection isn't always obvious — but it's real.
- Some treatments that save lives can also **change hormone levels**, **reduce calcium absorption**, or **slow bone rebuilding.**
- That doesn't mean osteoporosis is inevitable — it just means your bone health needs extra attention and care.

1. Cancer Treatments and Bone Loss

Hormone-Related Cancers: Cancers that depend on hormones — such as **breast, prostate, or ovarian cancer** — are most likely to affect bone density, mainly because treatments often *reduce or block hormones that protect bones.*

For Women (and rarely Men): Breast Cancer

- Treatments like **aromatase inhibitors** (e.g., **Arimidex® [anastrozole]**, **Femara® [letrozole]**, **Aromasin® [exemestane]**) lower estrogen, which normally helps protect bone.
- **Chemotherapy** and **early menopause** caused by treatment can also accelerate bone loss.
- Long-term **steroid use** (often given to prevent nausea or allergic reactions) further increases risk.

What Helps:

- DEXA scans before and during treatment
- Calcium (1,200 mg/day) and vitamin D_3 (800–1,000 IU/day)
- Weight-bearing exercise (walking, resistance training)
- Bisphosphonates or **Denosumab (Prolia®)** — often used to preserve bone and reduce fracture risk

What to Avoid:

- **Hormone replacement therapy (HRT)** — not recommended for most breast cancer survivors, as it may increase recurrence risk

For Men: Prostate Cancer

- **Androgen deprivation therapy (ADT)** — drugs like **Lupron® (leuprolide)** or **Zoladex® (goserelin)** — lowers testosterone, which normally supports bone building.
- Long-term use can cause significant bone loss and higher fracture risk.

What Helps:

- Calcium and vitamin D_3
- Strength and balance exercises
- **Bisphosphonates (Reclast®, Fosamax®)** or **Denosumab (Prolia®)** — both approved to protect bone during ADT
- Regular bone density scans (usually every 1–2 years)

Other Cancer Treatments That Can Affect Bone Health

- **Chemotherapy:** Can interfere with hormones, appetite, and nutrient absorption.
- **Radiation therapy:** May reduce blood flow to bone or damage nearby tissues.
- **Bone marrow transplant:** Can cause rapid bone loss due to steroids or immune changes.
- **Medications for multiple myeloma or leukemia:** Sometimes cause calcium and vitamin D imbalance.

2. Conditions That Mimic or Worsen Osteoporosis

Some health conditions naturally increase bone loss or make bones more fragile:

Condition	How It Affects Bone
Thyroid disease	Too much thyroid hormone speeds bone loss.
Parathyroid disease	Pulls calcium out of bones and raises blood calcium levels.
Celiac disease or Crohn's disease	Makes it harder to absorb calcium and vitamin D.
Rheumatoid arthritis	Inflammation and steroid use both weaken bone.
Chronic kidney disease	Interferes with vitamin D and calcium balance.
Diabetes	May reduce bone quality and healing ability.

Tip: If you have any of these conditions, your provider may tailor your medication and supplement plan differently — for example, lowering your calcium dose if your parathyroid or kidney function is affected.

3. Which Bone Medications Are Safe After Cancer

Medication Type	Usually Safe for Cancer Survivors	Caution / Avoid
Bisphosphonates (Fosamax®, Reclast®)	✔ Safe and often used to prevent cancer-related bone loss	Use with dental monitoring — rare risk of jaw bone injury
Denosumab (Prolia®)	✔ Very effective in cancer-related bone loss	Must continue on schedule; stopping suddenly causes rebound bone loss
Anabolic agents (Forteo®, Tymlos®)	▲ *Avoid if you've had bone cancer or radiation to bones*	Can raise bone formation, but not used in cancer-related bone disease
Romosozumab (Evenity®)	✔ Safe in most people; discuss if you have heart disease	Used for severe osteoporosis or multiple fractures
Hormone therapy (estrogen, Evista®)	▲ Usually *not* used in hormone-sensitive cancers	May raise recurrence risk; always discuss with oncology team
Calcitonin (Miacalcin®)	✔ Generally safe but less effective	Short-term use only for spine fracture pain

- Always check with your **oncologist or endocrinologist** before starting or stopping any bone medication.
- The right choice depends on your cancer history, treatment type, and current lab results.

4. Bone-Healthy Living During and After Cancer Treatment

- **Nutrition:** Eat balanced meals with calcium-rich foods (milk, yogurt, leafy greens, beans, fortified non-dairy options).
- **Vitamin D_3:** Take supplements if blood levels are low — sunlight may not be enough during treatment.
- **Exercise:** Gentle weight-bearing exercise, yoga, or tai chi can reduce fatigue and strengthen bones.
- **Avoid smoking and limit alcohol** — both interfere with bone repair and healing.
- **Hydration:** Helps prevent constipation (especially when taking calcium supplements).

---

5. Questions to Ask Your Provider

- ☐ Am I at risk for bone loss due to my cancer treatment or health condition? ______
- ☐ Which bone medications are safe for me? ______

______

- ☐ How often should I have a bone density scan? ______

______

- ☐ Should I be taking calcium and vitamin D, and how much?

______

- ☐ Are there exercises or safety precautions I should follow?

______

- ☐ Should I see an endocrinologist or a bone health specialist?

______

The Takeaway

- Cancer treatments can affect your bones — but with early testing, the right medication, and healthy daily habits, you can rebuild and protect your strength.
- Bone health is part of your recovery, not separate from it.

Section 14

Monitoring, Follow-Up, and Re-Testing

Staying on Track With Your Bone Health Plan

Why Follow-Up Is Important

- Bone health doesn't change overnight — it changes slowly, over months or years.
- That's why regular check-ins and follow-up testing are key to making sure your plan is working.

Your provider will use this information to see if:

- Your medications are helping your bones stay strong
- Your supplements and nutrition are balanced
- Any side effects or new health issues need attention

Think of bone health like a long-term project — checking progress along the way keeps you moving in the right direction.

---

1. Bone Density Scans (DEXA or Other Imaging)

Your bone density scan (DEXA) is the main way your provider tracks changes in bone strength.

What Your Provider Looks For:

- Has your T-score stayed the same, improved, or decreased?
- Are there signs that medication is working?
- Do any areas (like your spine or hips) show new weakness?

When to Repeat:

- There's no one-size-fits-all schedule.

The right timing depends on:

- Your age and overall health
- Whether you're on medication — and which type
- If you've had any new fractures or falls
- Whether your lab results or symptoms have changed*
- Some people re-test sooner; others wait longer.
- Your medical provider will decide what makes sense for you — *don't skip or delay follow-ups without discussing it first.*

---

2. Blood Work and Lab Monitoring

Many people will need periodic blood tests to check:

- Calcium and vitamin D levels — to be sure supplements are helping, not harming
- Kidney and liver function — especially if taking bisphosphonates or other long-term medications
- Parathyroid or thyroid hormones — if these conditions are contributing to bone loss
- Bone turnover markers (like CTX or NTX) — to measure how fast bone is breaking down

Your provider may also repeat other labs if your medication changes or if a new medical issue arises.

---

3. Medication Check-Ins 💊

Whether you take oral, injectable, or IV treatments, it's important to keep your follow-up appointments so your provider can:

- Make sure you're not missing doses
- Check for side effects or dental issues (especially with bisphosphonates or Prolia®)
- Review any changes in pain, movement, or energy
- Decide when or if to take a "medication holiday"

Never stop a bone medication suddenly without a replacement plan — especially if you take Denosumab (Prolia®), since stopping abruptly can cause rapid bone loss.

---

4. Reassessing Risk

- Bone health changes with life changes.

Each year, your provider may ask about:

- Any new falls or fractures
- New medications or health diagnoses
- Weight or hormone changes
- Changes in balance, strength, or vision
- Lifestyle habits (smoking, exercise, or alcohol use)

Even small shifts in these areas can affect your fracture risk — and your care plan may be adjusted accordingly.

---

5. Self-Monitoring Between Visits

You can also track your own progress by noting:

- Energy and balance improvements
- Less back or joint pain
- How confident you feel moving or walking
- Daily supplement or exercise consistency

Keep a small **"Bone Health Journal"** to jot down what's working well and what questions to bring to your next visit.

---

6. When to Call Your Provider Sooner

Reach out to your medical provider if you:

- Have sudden or new back pain (possible compression fracture)
- Lose more than an inch of height
- Have a new fall, even if you didn't break anything
- Notice unusual thigh or jaw pain (especially if on bisphosphonates)
- Develop numbness, weakness, or severe fatigue

Early communication can help catch problems before they become serious.

Red-Flag List — Call Promptly

- New back pain that doesn't go away
- New thigh or groin pain
- Trouble swallowing after a bone pill
- Missed Prolia® or Reclast® appointment
- Two or more near-falls in one week
  Early calls = early fixes.

Navigating Your Care Team and Resources

Keeping bones strong often takes a team:

Team Member	How They Help
Primary Care Provider	Coordinates your overall plan and orders DEXA scans.
Endocrinologist	Specializes in hormone and metabolism causes of bone loss.
Orthopedic Specialist	Manages fractures and surgical treatments. Some specialize in bone health also
Physical Therapist	Builds strength, balance, and safe movement after fracture.
Occupational Therapist	Teaches ways to do daily tasks safely and prevent falls.
Dietitian	Designs meal plans for calcium, vitamin D, and protein.
Pharmacist	Checks drug interactions and reminds you about refills.

Social Worker / Case Manager	Finds community resources and financial assistance.

Programs and Support

- In 2025, Medicare covers DEXA scans every 2 years for qualified patients.
- Local senior centers often offer free balance classes or fall-proofing workshops.
- The Bone Health & Osteoporosis Foundation (www.bonehealthandosteoporosis.org)
- NIH (NIAMS) – “Exercise for Your Bone Health”
- Mayo Clinic and Cleveland Clinic – patient handouts on osteoporosis care.

Asking for help is a sign of strength — not weakness.

- These resources exist to keep you safe, independent, and supported.

🖤 Financial and Community Support Resources

Because Strong Bones Shouldn’t Depend on Your Wallet

Taking care of your bones shouldn’t cause financial stress. Many national and local programs can help cover testing, medications, and safety equipment.

Insurance and Testing

- **Medicare Part B** – covers a bone density (DEXA) scan every 2 years for qualified patients, or sooner if medically necessary.
- **Medicare Advantage & Private Plans** – may include extra wellness visits or preventive benefits; ask about "bone health screening" coverage.
- **Medicare Extra Help / Medicaid** – may lower the cost of prescriptions like Prolia®, Fosamax®, or Reclast®.
- **Patient-Assistance Programs** – manufacturers such as Amgen (Prolia®), Novartis (Reclast®), and Lilly (Forteo®) offer financial-help applications on their websites.

Community and Non-Profit Resources

- **Bone Health & Osteoporosis Foundation (BHOF)**
  Website: www.bonehealthandosteoporosis.org
  Free exercise handouts, educational videos, and support groups.
- **NIAMS (National Institute of Arthritis and Musculoskeletal and Skin Diseases)**
  Offers printable brochures and community education on safe exercise.
- **YMCA & Local Senior Centers**
  Many locations offer low-cost "Silver Sneakers" or balance classes to prevent falls.

- **Area Agencies on Aging**
 County offices that connect older adults to transportation, home-safety equipment, and nutrition programs. Find yours at www.eldercare.acl.gov.

- **Meals on Wheels**
 Delivers balanced meals rich in calcium and protein to homebound adults.

- **Local Health Departments**
 May lend walkers, shower chairs, or grab bars for temporary use.

Helpful Tips

- Your provider includes "osteoporosis diagnosis" on referrals or prescriptions — it can qualify you for additional services.

- Keep receipts for safety items (grab bars, shower chair); some insurance or HSA accounts will reimburse them.

- Bring a friend or family member to help complete financial-aid forms — extra eyes make the process easier.

Remember: help is out there, and using these resources is part of good self-care.
You've already taken the most important step — learning how to protect your bones.

Key Takeaways

- Monitoring bone health isn't about chasing numbers — it's about protecting your quality of life.
- How often you need scans or labs will depend on *you* — your medical history, your treatment, and your provider's guidance.
- Stay involved, stay informed, and keep the conversation open.

Your bones — and your future mobility — are worth it.

Section 15

Living Confidently With Osteoporosis

Hope, Strength, and the Power of Everyday Choices

You Are Not Your Diagnosis

- Hearing the word *osteoporosis* can feel overwhelming — like your bones have betrayed you.

But here's the truth: **you are not your diagnosis.**

- You are a whole person — body, mind, and spirit — with many ways to protect your health and live fully.
- Osteoporosis doesn't mean weakness or limitation.
- It means awareness — and opportunity.
- It means paying attention to what your body needs and giving it the care it deserves.

---

1. Shifting the Mindset

- Instead of thinking: "I'm getting older — I'm falling apart," → try thinking, "I'm getting wiser — and I'm learning to take care of myself in new ways."
- Every time you stretch, lift, walk, eat well, or rest, you're building strength.
- Each small choice supports your bones, your muscles, and your confidence.

Mindful tip:

- When you take your supplements or go for a walk, say to yourself: "I'm investing in my future strength."
- It turns a routine into an act of self-care.

---

2. Practicing Mindfulness for Stronger Living

- Mindfulness isn't just for stress — it also helps your body heal and rebuild.
- When your mind is calm, your muscles relax, your breathing deepens, and your body absorbs nutrients and rests more efficiently.

Simple ways to practice mindfulness:

- **Breathe deeply** — in through your nose, out through your mouth — when you start your day.
- **Eat slowly**, noticing the flavors and textures of bone-friendly foods.
- **Walk with awareness** — feel each step, the ground beneath your feet, and the rhythm of your breath.
- **Let go of fear** by focusing on what's in your control right now.

You don't have to meditate for hours — mindfulness is simply paying attention, with kindness, to this moment.

---

3. Building Emotional Strength Alongside Bone Strength 💪

- It's normal to feel frustrated, especially if you've had a fracture or need to change your routine.
- But emotional resilience — the ability to adapt, cope, and bounce back — is a skill you can practice every day.

Try This:

- Keep a **gratitude list** of three things you appreciate daily.
- Celebrate progress — even small ones like walking a few minutes longer or choosing water instead of soda.
- Stay connected — talk to friends, join support groups, or attend local osteoporosis events.

Remember: it's okay to ask for help — from family, therapists, or your healthcare team.

- Strong bones help you stand tall — but a strong spirit keeps you moving forward.

---

4. Creating a Bone-Healthy Lifestyle You Enjoy

- Bone health isn't about strict rules — it's about balance and joy.
- You can nourish your body *and* live fully.

A few uplifting habits:

- **Move every day:** Find something fun — dancing, gardening, walking your dog, or swimming.
- **Eat with purpose:** Focus on colorful, nourishing foods that fuel both body and mind.
- **Get sunshine:** A few minutes outdoors boosts vitamin D and mood.
- **Sleep well:** Rest is when bones and muscles repair themselves.
- **Protect your peace:** Limit stress where possible. Stress hormones can weaken bones over time.

---

5. A Note on Comparison

- It's easy to compare yourself to how you used to move or what others can do.

But your journey is *yours alone.*

- Healing happens at your own pace — and progress is still progress, even when it's quiet or slow.

- Focus on consistency, not perfection.
- Each day that you move, eat well, rest, and care for yourself — that's a victory.

---

6. A Guided Moment of Mindfulness

- Let's end this chapter — and this book — with a brief mindfulness practice you can return to anytime.

Find a quiet space.

- Sit or stand tall, with your spine straight but relaxed.
- Take a deep breath in…
- and slowly let it go.

Feel your feet rooted to the ground.

- Imagine your bones as strong, flexible supports — steady, but never brittle.
- With each breath, picture light and warmth filling your body from head to toe.
- Your breath is strength.
- Your stillness is stability.
- Your awareness is healing.

When you're ready, open your eyes and carry that calm strength with you into your day.

Remember This

- Osteoporosis is not an ending — it's a reminder to live with more awareness, care, and strength.
- Every choice you make — every meal, every step, every breath — can build a healthier, more confident you.
- You have the tools.
- You have the knowledge.
- You have the power to protect your bones — and your future.

Fall Prevention & Home Safety 🪑 *(Most of these are low-cost and easy to install.)*

Bathroom:

- Grab bars (stainless or suction-based)
- Nonslip bath mats
- Shower chair or bench
- Raised toilet seat with arms
- Handheld showerhead

Bedroom:

- Bedside lamp with touch control
- Motion-sensor nightlights
- Bed rail assist handle
- Floor-to-ceiling transfer pole (for stability when standing)

Living Areas:

- Rug grippers or nonslip pads
- Cord management clips
- Reach/grabber tool (32-inch length)
- Recliner risers (for easier standing)

Footwear & Safety:

- Nonslip house shoes or socks with grips
- Orthopedic walking shoes
- Fall alert or medical alert pendant (for higher-risk individuals)

Mindfulness & Comfort

Aromatherapy diffuser with calming essential oils

- Weighted blanket (for relaxation)
- Guided meditation CDs or apps (search *"Mindfulness for Seniors"*)
- Journals or gratitude notebooks
- Ergonomic chair cushion or lumbar support

Educational & Support Resources

- *Mayo Clinic Guide to Bone Health*
- *Strong Women, Strong Bones* by Miriam Nelson
- *The Whole-Body Approach to Osteoporosis* by R. Keith McCormick, DC
- *Yoga for Osteoporosis* (book by Loren Fishman, MD)
- *Osteoporosis Canada – Too Fit To Fall or Fracture* (PDF)

Bone Health Trackers & Checklists

Medication Tracker

Medication	Dose	How often	Notes
1)			
2)			
3)			
4)			
5)			

Bone Care Checklist

☐ Took calcium and vitamin D

☐ 30 minutes of activity

☐ Ate a protein food

☐ Drank water

☐ Practiced good posture

Bone Density and Lab Log

Date	Test Type	Result (T-score or Lab)	Next Due Date
1)			
2)			
3)			
4)			
5)			
6)			
7)			
8)			
9)			
10)			

Use these pages to stay organized and celebrate progress over time.

GLOSSARY

A

Anabolic medications—Drugs that help the body build new bone by stimulating bone-forming cells

Anemia—A condition where you don't have enough red blood cells to carry oxygen through your body

Arthritis—Inflammation of the joints that causes pain, stiffness, or swelling

B

Balance—The ability to keep your body stable and upright while moving or standing still

Bisphosphonates—Medications that slow bone loss by reducing the breakdown of bone cells

Bone density—A measure of how much mineral content, mainly calcium, is in your bones

Bone mineral density (BMD)—The measurement obtained from a DEXA scan to assess bone strength

C

Calcitonin—A hormone that helps regulate calcium and can be used as a nasal spray for bone pain

Calcium—A mineral essential for building and maintaining strong bones and teeth

Celiac disease—An autoimmune condition that prevents the body from absorbing nutrients properly when gluten is eaten

Collagen—A protein that provides structure and flexibility to bone and connective tissues

Compression fracture—A collapse or break in one of the spinal bones, often caused by osteoporosis

D

DEXA scan—A painless test that measures bone density using low-dose X-rays

Denosumab—A medication that slows bone loss by blocking the cells that break down bone

Dietary supplements—Vitamins, minerals, or nutrients taken to support health in addition to food

Dual-energy X-ray absorptiometry—The full name for the DEXA scan used to diagnose osteoporosis

E

Estrogen—A female hormone that helps maintain bone density; levels drop after menopause

Evenity—A brand name for romosozumab, a medication that helps build bone and reduce fracture risk

Exercise—Physical activity that strengthens bones, muscles, and balance

F

Fall prevention—Steps taken to reduce the risk of falling and fracturing bones

Forteo—A brand name for teriparatide, an anabolic medication that helps build bone

Fracture—A break in a bone

G

Glucocorticoids—A type of steroid medication that can cause bone loss when used long term

Grab bars—Handles installed in bathrooms or near stairs to help prevent falls

H

Hormone replacement therapy (HRT)—A treatment that replaces estrogen after menopause but is not recommended for all women

Hyperthyroidism—A condition in which the thyroid gland is overactive, causing bone loss

Hypocalcemia—Low calcium levels in the blood that can affect muscle and bone function

I

Ionized calcium—The active form of calcium in the blood that your body can use directly

IV infusion—Delivery of medication through a vein

J

Joint—The point where two bones meet and allow movement

K

Kyphoplasty—A minimally invasive procedure to repair a spinal compression fracture

L

Lab tests—Blood or urine tests used to check for vitamin, hormone, or mineral problems that affect bones

Low bone mass—Bone density that is lower than normal but not yet osteoporosis

M

Magnesium—A mineral that helps your body use calcium and vitamin D effectively

Menopause—The natural end of menstrual cycles that causes a drop in estrogen and increased bone loss

Miacalcin—A brand name for calcitonin used to help with bone pain or fractures

Mindfulness—The practice of paying attention to the present moment with calm and awareness

N

Nutrition—The process of eating and absorbing nutrients needed for body and bone health

O

Occupational therapy—A healthcare service that teaches safer ways to perform daily activities after illness or injury

Osteoblast—A type of bone cell that builds new bone tissue

Osteoclast—A type of bone cell that breaks down old bone tissue

Osteopenia—A condition where bone density is lower than normal but not as severe as osteoporosis

Osteoporosis—A condition where bones become weak and brittle, increasing the risk of fracture

P

Parathyroid hormone (PTH)—A hormone that regulates calcium levels in the body

Physical therapy—Exercise and movement training to improve strength, balance, and mobility

Prolia—A brand name for denosumab, a medication that helps prevent bone loss

Protein—A nutrient that supports muscle, bone, and tissue repair

R

Raloxifene—A medication that acts like estrogen in bones but not in other tissues

Reclast—A brand name for zoledronic acid, a bisphosphonate given as a yearly IV infusion

Resistance training—Exercise that uses weights or resistance bands to strengthen muscles and bones

Romosozumab—A medication that helps build new bone and reduce fractures

S

SERMs—Selective estrogen receptor modulators, a class of medications that mimic estrogen in bone

Sodium—A mineral found in salt; too much can increase calcium loss from bones

Steroids—Medications that reduce inflammation but can weaken bone over time

Supplement—A product that provides vitamins or minerals to fill gaps in your diet

T

Teriparatide—A medication that stimulates bone growth and reduces fracture risk

Thyroid—A gland in the neck that controls metabolism and affects bone turnover

T-score—A measurement from the DEXA scan comparing your bone density to that of a healthy young adult

V

Vertebroplasty—A procedure that injects cement into a spinal bone to relieve pain from a compression fracture

Vitamin D—A vitamin that helps your body absorb calcium and build strong bones

W

Weight-bearing exercise—Activity that makes your bones work against gravity, like walking or dancing

Z

Zoledronic acid—A medication given through an IV once a year to strengthen bones

---

AUTHOR NOTE

As a Physician Assistant and educator, my goal has always been to make medical information clear, compassionate, and useful. *Osteoporosis 101: A Patient's Complete Guide to Bone Health, Prevention, and Treatment* was written to help people understand that bone loss is not a sentence—it's a signal. It's a reminder that we can take control of our health at any age through knowledge, movement, nutrition, and care.

This book joins my growing patient education series, which includes *Breast Cancer 101: A Complete Guide for Patients and Their Families – From Diagnosis to Healing* and *Menopause 101: What Every Husband Should Know About the Change.* Both are also available in Spanish editions (*Cáncer de Mama 101* and *Menopausia 101*) to help reach the Spanish-speaking community with accessible, trustworthy medical information.

Each book in this series is designed for real people—patients, families, and caregivers—who deserve to understand what's happening inside their bodies without feeling overwhelmed by medical jargon. If these books bring you comfort, clarity, or confidence during your healthcare journey, then they have done their job.

Thank you for reading and for taking an active role in your health. You are stronger than you think—inside and out.

—*Stacie PA-C*
Duke Residency Trained Physician Assistant
Founder, **Medical Things Explained**
Author of the *Patient Education 101 Series*

QUICK INDEX

More Helpful Books by Stacie the PA

Clear, compassionate, and practical guides written by a medical provider who cares.

Kidney Stones 101
A clear guide to causes, treatments, and prevention strategies.

Hypertension 101
Understand high blood pressure and how to manage it — simply.

Knee Pain 101
From anatomy to treatment options, a complete patient reference.

Hip Pain 101
Everything you need to know about hip pain, diagnosis, and care.

Shoulder Pain 101
An easy-to-follow guide to common shoulder problems and solutions.

Neck Pain 101
An easy-to-follow guide to spine-related neck pain, diagnosis, and treatment options.

Pneumonia 101
Learn the basics of prevention, symptoms, and recovery.

Gout 101
Practical answers about causes, flares, and long-term care.

Diverticulosis 101
Understand symptoms, triggers, and treatment of this common digestive condition.

Breast Cancer 101: A Patient's Complete Guide to Symptoms, Treatments, and Prevention
A compassionate, evidence-based guide for patients, survivors,

and caregivers — covering everything from diagnosis to recovery and long-term wellness.

🎗 **Cáncer de Mama 101: Guía Completa para Pacientes**
The Spanish-language edition of *Breast Cancer 101* — designed to serve North American Spanish-speaking patients and families with the same supportive, educational approach.

✸ **Menopause 101: What Every Husband Should Know About the Change.**

✸ **Coming soon Menopause 101 in Spanish, and Back Pain 101:** A complete guide to understanding, treating, and preventing back pain.

🌐 Stay Connected

Follow for updates, educational content, and patient-friendly health tips:

Website: https://staciethepa.com/
Amazon Author Page: Stacie the PA on Amazon
Social: @StacieThePA

Affiliate Note

Some of the links on my website or author page may be affiliate links. This means I may earn a small commission if you purchase through them — at no additional cost to you.
These proceeds help fund the creation of more patient-education books, toolkits, and free online resources.

Thank you for your support!

Made in the USA
Monee, IL
06 June 2026

51898921R00085